TYPE 2 AUTOIMMUNE HEPATITIS COOKBOOK

Delicious and Nutritious Recipes to Manage the Liver and Support Healthy Lifestyle

Sonia Emmason

Copyright © 2023 by Sonia Emmason

All rights reserved. No part of this publication may be reproduced, distributed, or transmitted in any form or by any means, including photocopying, recording, or other electronic or mechanical methods, without the prior written permission of the publisher, except in the case of brief quotations embodied in critical reviews and certain other noncommercial uses permitted by copyright law.

CHAPTER 1

Type 2 autoimmune hepatitis (AIH) is a chronic liver disease characterized by inflammation and damage to liver cells due to an autoimmune response. This means that the immune system mistakenly attacks the liver, leading to inflammation and scarring. Over time, this can lead to liver cirrhosis and liver failure. While the exact cause of type 2 AIH is not fully understood, it is believed to be a combination of genetic and environmental factors.

While there is no cure for type 2 AIH, it can be managed through medication and lifestyle changes. One of the key lifestyle changes that can help manage the symptoms of type 2 AIH is a healthy diet.

A healthy diet for type 2 AIH should focus on reducing inflammation in the liver and providing essential nutrients to support liver function. This means avoiding foods that can cause further damage to the liver, such as processed foods, high-fat foods and alcohol. Instead, the diet should include whole, nutrient-dense foods that are rich in antioxidants and anti-inflammatory compounds.

One of the key nutrients that is important for liver health is protein. Protein is essential for the repair and regeneration of liver cells, and can also help reduce inflammation in the liver. Good sources of protein for a type 2 AIH diet include lean meats, fish, eggs, beans, and legumes.

In addition to protein, a type 2 AIH diet should also include plenty of fruits and vegetables. These foods are rich in vitamins, minerals, and antioxidants, which can help reduce inflammation in the liver and support overall liver function. Some good choices include leafy greens, berries, citrus fruits, and cruciferous vegetables like broccoli and cauliflower.

Fiber is another important nutrient for a type 2 AIH diet. Fiber helps to keep the digestive system healthy, which is important for overall liver health. Good sources of fiber include whole grains, fruits, vegetables, and legumes.

Omega-3 fatty acids are also beneficial for type 2 AIH. These healthy fats can help reduce inflammation in the liver and support overall liver function. Good sources of omega-3 fatty acids include fatty fish like salmon, sardines, and mackerel, as well as chia seeds, flaxseeds, and walnuts.

On the other hand, there are certain foods that should be avoided or limited in a type 2 AIH diet. These include processed foods, high-fat foods, and alcohol. Processed foods are often high in sugar, salt, and unhealthy fats, all of which can contribute to inflammation and liver damage. High-fat foods can also be hard for the liver to process, which can further strain an already compromised liver. Alcohol, in particular, is toxic to the liver and can cause further damage.

In addition to making dietary changes, it is also important to maintain a healthy weight and engage in regular exercise. Being overweight or obese can increase the risk of liver damage in type 2 AIH, so maintaining a healthy weight can help reduce this risk.

Exercise is also important for overall liver health, as it can help reduce inflammation and improve liver function.

Overall, a healthy diet is an important component of managing type 2 autoimmune hepatitis. By focusing on whole, nutrient-dense foods and avoiding processed foods, high-fat foods, and alcohol, it is possible to support liver function and reduce inflammation in the liver. With the right diet and lifestyle changes, it is possible to manage the symptoms of type 2 AIH and improve overall liver health.

CHAPTER 2

2.1 CAUSES OF TYPE 2 AUTOIMMUNE HEPATITIS

The exact cause of type 2 autoimmune hepatitis (AIH) is not fully understood. However, it is believed to be a combination of genetic and environmental factors that trigger an autoimmune response in the liver.

Genetic factors may play a role in the development of type 2 AIH, as it has been found to run in families. Some studies have identified specific genetic variations that may increase the risk of developing the condition.

Environmental factors may also contribute to the development of type 2 AIH. These factors may include exposure to toxins, infections, and certain medications. Some studies suggest that type 2 AIH may be triggered by a viral infection, such as hepatitis C or Epstein-Barr virus.

It is important to note that while these factors may increase the risk of developing type 2 AIH, not everyone who is exposed to these factors will develop the condition. Other factors, such as a person's immune system and overall health, may also play a role in the development of type 2 AIH.

Overall, the exact causes of type 2 AIH are still not fully understood, and more research is needed to determine the underlying mechanisms of the condition.

2.2 SYMPTOMS OF TYPE 2 AUTOIMMUNE HEPATITIS

Type 2 autoimmune hepatitis (AIH) is a chronic liver disease that can cause a range of symptoms. The severity of symptoms can vary from person to person, and some people may not experience any symptoms at all. However, common symptoms of type 2 AIH may include:

1. **Fatigue:** Many people with type 2 AIH experience fatigue, which can range from mild to severe.

2. **Abdominal Discomfort:** Some people may experience abdominal pain, bloating, or discomfort.

3. **Joint Pain:** Joint pain and stiffness may occur in some people with type 2 AIH.

4. **Jaundice:** Jaundice is a yellowing of the skin and eyes that can occur when the liver is not functioning properly.

5. **Itching:** Itching can occur when the liver is not able to process bile properly.

6. **Nausea and Vomiting:** Some people may experience nausea and vomiting, particularly in the early stages of the disease.

7. **Loss of Appetite:** Loss of appetite can occur in some people with type 2 AIH.

8. **Spider Angiomas:** Spider angiomas are small, spider-like blood vessels that can appear on the skin.

9. **Enlarged Liver and Spleen:** In some cases, the liver and spleen may become enlarged.

It is important to note that not everyone with type 2 AIH will experience all of these symptoms, and some people may not experience any symptoms at all. If you are experiencing any of these symptoms, it is important to see a healthcare provider for an evaluation and proper diagnosis. Early diagnosis and treatment can help prevent further liver damage and improve outcomes.

2.3 DIAGNOSIS OF TYPE 2 AUTOIMMUNE HEPATITIS

The diagnosis of type 2 autoimmune hepatitis (AIH) involves several steps, including a thorough medical history, physical examination, and various laboratory tests. If a healthcare provider suspects that a person may have type 2 AIH, they may refer the person to a specialist, such as a gastroenterologist or hepatologist for further evaluation and treatment.

The following are some of the tests and procedures that may be used to diagnose type 2 AIH:

1. **Blood Tests:** Blood tests can be used to check for the presence of certain antibodies, such as anti-

LKM-1 and anti-LC-1, which are associated with type 2 AIH. Other blood tests, such as liver function tests, can help evaluate how well the liver is functioning.

2. **Imaging Tests:** Imaging tests, such as ultrasound, CT scan, or MRI, can be used to evaluate the liver for signs of damage or inflammation.

3. **Liver Biopsy:** A liver biopsy involves taking a small sample of tissue from the liver for examination under a microscope. This can help confirm the diagnosis of type 2 AIH and assess the severity of liver damage.

4. **Other Tests:** Other tests, such as an endoscopy or colonoscopy, may be performed to evaluate the digestive tract for signs of inflammation or damage.

It is important to note that the diagnosis of type 2 AIH can be challenging, as the condition can mimic other liver diseases. For this reason, it is important to have a thorough evaluation by a healthcare provider who specializes in liver diseases. Early diagnosis and treatment can help prevent further liver damage and improve outcomes for people with type 2 AIH.

CHAPTER 3

3.0 NUTRITION AND DIET

3.1 HEALTHY EATING

For people with type 2 autoimmune hepatitis (AIH), adopting a healthy eating plan can help support liver health and overall well-being. A healthy eating plan for people with type 2 AIH should focus on nutrient-dense foods that provide essential vitamins and minerals, while limiting foods that may contribute to liver damage or inflammation.

Here are some tips for healthy eating with type 2 AIH:

1. **Eat a Variety of Fruits and Vegetables:** Fruits and vegetables are rich in vitamins, minerals, and antioxidants that can help support liver health. Aim to include a variety of colors and types of fruits and vegetables in your diet.

2. **Choose Whole Grains:** Whole grains, such as brown rice, quinoa, and whole wheat bread, are

rich in fiber and nutrients that can help support digestive health.

3. **Include Lean Protein Sources:** Lean protein sources, such as chicken, fish, tofu, and beans, can provide essential amino acids without contributing excess fat or cholesterol.

4. **Limit Saturated and Trans Fats:** Saturated and trans fats can contribute to liver damage and inflammation. Limit foods that are high in saturated and trans fats, such as fatty meats, fried foods, and baked foods.

5. **Avoid Processed Foods:** Processed foods, such as fast food and packaged snacks, often contain high levels of salt, sugar, and unhealthy fats that can contribute to inflammation and other health problems.

6. **Limit Alcohol Intake:** Alcohol can be particularly damaging to the liver in people with type 2 AIH. It is important to limit or avoid alcohol completely.

7. **Stay Hydrated:** Drinking plenty of water and other fluids can help support liver function and overall health.

It is important to work with a healthcare provider to develop a personalized eating plan that meets your individual needs and health goals. Additionally, if you are taking any medications for type 2 AIH, it is important to discuss potential interactions with certain foods or supplements with your healthcare provider.

3.2 FOODS TO AVOID

For people with type 2 autoimmune hepatitis (AIH), certain foods can contribute to liver damage or inflammation and should be avoided or limited. It is important to note that everyone's body may react differently to certain foods, so it is essential to work with a healthcare provider to develop a personalized eating plan that meets your individual needs and health goals.

Here are some foods and beverages to avoid or limit with type 2 AIH:

1. **Alcohol:** Alcohol can be particularly damaging to the liver in people with type 2 AIH. It is important to limit or avoid alcohol completely.

2. **Processed Foods:** Processed foods, such as fast food, frozen meals and packaged snacks, often contain high levels of salt, sugar and unhealthy fats that can contribute to inflammation and other health problems.

3. **Fried Foods:** Fried foods, such as French fries and fried chicken, can be high in unhealthy fats and can contribute to inflammation and liver damage.

4. **Fatty Meats:** Fatty meats, such as beef, pork, and lamb, can be high in saturated and trans fats, which can contribute to inflammation and liver damage.

5. **High-Sugar Foods and Beverages:** Foods and beverages that are high in sugar such as soda, candy and pastries can contribute to inflammation and liver damage.

6. **High-Salt Foods:** Foods that are high in salt, such as processed meats and canned soups, can contribute to fluid retention and liver damage.

7. **Some Dietary Supplements:** Some dietary supplements, such as high doses of vitamin A and

iron, can be harmful to the liver in people with type 2 AIH. It is important to discuss potential interactions with certain supplements with your healthcare provider.

It is important to note that the foods listed above are not necessarily harmful to everyone, but may be problematic for some people with type 2 AIH. Additionally, certain foods may interact with medications used to treat type 2 AIH, so it is essential to work closely with a healthcare provider to ensure that your eating plan supports your liver health and overall well-being.

3.3 THE ROLE OF SUPPLEMENTS

Supplements can be a useful addition to a healthy eating plan for people with type 2 autoimmune hepatitis (AIH). However, it is important to note that supplements should not be used as a substitute for a balanced diet or medication prescribed by a healthcare provider. Additionally, supplements can interact with medications used to treat type 2 AIH.

Here are some supplements that may be beneficial for people with type 2 AIH:

1. **Omega-3 Fatty Acids:** Omega-3 fatty acids, found in fatty fish, flaxseed, and chia seeds, have anti-inflammatory properties that can help reduce inflammation in the liver. Some people with type 2 AIH may benefit from taking omega-3 supplements, but it is important to discuss the appropriate dose with a healthcare provider.

2. **Vitamin D:** Vitamin D plays a role in immune system function and may help reduce inflammation in the liver. Some people with type 2 AIH may have low levels of vitamin D, and may benefit from taking supplements to support their overall health.

3. **Milk Thistle:** Milk thistle is an herbal supplement that has been used for centuries to support liver health. Some studies have suggested that milk thistle may have anti-inflammatory properties and may help protect the liver from damage. However, more research is needed to fully

understand the potential benefits of milk thistle for people with type 2 AIH.

4. **N-acetylcysteine (NAC):** NAC is a supplement that may help reduce inflammation in the liver and protect against oxidative stress. Some studies have suggested that NAC may be beneficial for people with liver diseases, including AIH, but more research is needed to fully understand the potential benefits and appropriate dosing.

5. **Probiotics:** Probiotics are live bacteria and yeasts that can help support digestive health. Some studies have suggested that probiotics may have anti-inflammatory properties and may help reduce liver inflammation in people with AIH.

It is important to note that supplements should be used in conjunction with a healthy eating plan and medication prescribed by a healthcare provider. Additionally, it is essential to work with a healthcare provider to ensure that supplements are appropriate for your individual needs and health goals.

CHAPTER 4

4.0 HEALTHY RECIPES FOR TYPE 2 AUTOIMMUNE HEPATITIS

4.1 BREAKFAST RECIPES

1. Healthy Oatmeal Pancakes (30 minutes)

Ingredients:

-1 cup rolled oats

-1 cup plain Greek yogurt

-1 egg

-1/2 teaspoon baking powder

-1/2 teaspoon vanilla extract

-1/4 teaspoon ground cinnamon

Instructions:

1. In a medium bowl, combine oats, yogurt, egg, baking powder, vanilla extract, and cinnamon. Mix until the ingredients are well combined.

2. Heat a non-stick skillet over medium heat and lightly grease it with oil or butter.

3. Drop about 1/4 cup of the pancake batter onto the skillet and cook for 3-4 minutes per side, or until golden brown.

4. Serve with your favorite topping and enjoy.

Ingredients:

-1 banana, frozen

-1/2 cup rolled oats

-1/2 cup almond milk

-1 tablespoon honey

-1 tablespoon ground flaxseed

Instructions:

1. Place all ingredients in a blender.

2. Blend until the mixture is smooth and creamy.

3. Pour into a glass and enjoy.

Ingredients:

-1 sweet potato

-1 tablespoon olive oil

-Salt, to taste

-Pepper, to taste

-1/4 cup feta cheese

-1/4 cup sliced cherry tomatoes

-1/4 cup chopped spinach

Instructions:

1. Preheat the oven to 375F.

2. Cut the sweet potato into 1/4-inch thick slices.

3. Place the slices on a baking sheet lined with parchment paper and brush with olive oil.

4. Sprinkle with salt and pepper.

5. Bake for 12-15 minutes or until the sweet potato slices are lightly golden.

6. To assemble, top each slice with feta cheese, cherry tomatoes, and spinach.

7. Serve and enjoy.

Ingredients:

-1 sweet potato, diced

-1 tablespoon olive oil

-1 onion, diced

-1 bell pepper, diced

-1 garlic clove, minced

-2 eggs

-Salt, to taste

-Pepper, to taste

Instructions:

1. Heat the olive oil in a large skillet over medium heat.

2. Add the sweet potato, onion, bell pepper, and garlic and cook for 5-7 minutes or until vegetables are softened.

3. Make two wells in the vegetables and crack in the eggs.

4. Cover the skillet and cook for 3-4 minutes or until the eggs are cooked to your preference.

5. Season with salt and pepper.

6. Serve and enjoy.

Ingredients:

-1 tablespoon olive oil

-1 onion, diced

-3 garlic cloves, minced

-1/2 teaspoon dried oregano

-1 cup cherry tomatoes, halved

-2 cups baby spinach

-4 eggs

-Salt, to taste

-Pepper, to taste

Instructions:

1. Preheat the oven to 375F.

2. Heat the olive oil in a large skillet over medium heat.

3. Add the onion and garlic and cook for 3-4 minutes or until softened.

4. Add the oregano, cherry tomatoes, and spinach and cook for an additional 2 minutes or until the spinach is wilted.

5. Divide the mixture among four oven-safe ramekins.

6. Crack one egg into each ramekin and season with salt and pepper.

7. Place the ramekins on a baking sheet and bake for 10-12 minutes or until eggs are cooked to your preference.

8. Serve and enjoy.

Ingredients:

-2 slices whole wheat bread

-1/2 avocado, mashed

-1/4 teaspoon garlic powder

-1/4 teaspoon onion powder

-Salt, to taste

-Pepper, to taste

Instructions:

1. Toast the bread.

2. In a small bowl, mash the avocado with garlic powder, onion powder, salt, and pepper.

3. Spread the mashed avocado on the toast slices.

4. Serve and enjoy.

Ingredients:

-1/2 cup chia seeds

-1 cup almond milk

-1 tablespoon honey

-1 teaspoon vanilla extract

Instructions:

1. Place the chia seeds, almond milk, honey, and vanilla extract in a bowl and stir until combined.

2. Cover the bowl and place in the refrigerator for at least 4 hours or overnight.

3. Serve with your favorite toppings and enjoy.

Ingredients:

-2 eggs

-2 tablespoons chopped bell pepper

-2 tablespoons chopped onion

-1/4 cup shredded cheese

-1/4 cup black beans

-1 whole wheat tortilla

-Salt, to taste

-Pepper, to taste

Instructions:

1. Heat a small skillet over medium heat.

2. Add the eggs and scramble until they are cooked to your preference.

3. Add the bell pepper, onion, and black beans to the skillet and cook for an additional 3-4 minutes.

4. Place the scrambled egg mixture on the tortilla and top with cheese.

5. Season with salt and pepper.

6. Roll up the tortilla and enjoy.

Ingredients:

-1 cup plain Greek yogurt

-1/2 cup blueberries

-1/2 cup raspberries

-1/4 cup granola

Instructions:

1. Place 1/4 cup of Greek yogurt in the bottom of a glass.

2. Top with 1/4 cup of blueberries and 1/4 cup of raspberries.

3. Add 1/4 cup of granola.

4. Repeat the layering of yogurt, berries, and granola.

5. Serve and enjoy.

Ingredients:

-2 eggs

-1/4 avocado, mashed

-2 slices whole wheat bread

-Salt, to taste

-Pepper, to taste

Instructions:

1. Toast the bread.

2. Heat a small skillet over medium heat.

3. Add the eggs and scramble until they are cooked to your preference.

4. Spread the mashed avocado on the toast slices.

5. Top with the scrambled eggs.

6. Season with salt and pepper.

7. Serve and enjoy.

1. Salmon and Asparagus Bake (30 minutes)

Ingredients:

- 2 tablespoons olive oil

- 2 salmon fillets

- 2 cloves garlic, minced

- 1/2 teaspoon dried oregano

- 1/2 teaspoon dried thyme

- 1/2 teaspoon smoked paprika

- 1/4 teaspoon sea salt

- 1/4 teaspoon black pepper

- 1 bunch of asparagus, trimmed and cut into 1-inch pieces

- 2 tablespoons freshly squeezed lemon juice

- 2 tablespoons freshly chopped parsley

Instructions:

1. Preheat oven to 375 degrees F.

2. Heat oil in an oven-safe skillet over medium-high heat. Add salmon fillets and cook for 2 minutes per side, or until lightly browned.

3. Add garlic, oregano, thyme, paprika, salt, and pepper to the pan and cook for 1 minute, stirring often.

4. Add asparagus to the pan and cook for 3 minutes, stirring often.

5. Transfer skillet to preheated oven and bake for 15 minutes, or until salmon is cooked through and asparagus is tender.

6. Drizzle with lemon juice and sprinkle with parsley. Serve immediately.

2. Quinoa and Vegetable Bowl (25 minutes)

Ingredients:

- 2 tablespoons olive oil

- 1/2 cup uncooked quinoa

- 1 cup vegetable broth

- 1/2 red onion, diced

- 1 red bell pepper, diced

- 1 cup mushrooms, diced

- 2 cloves garlic, minced

- 1/2 teaspoon dried oregano

- 1/4 teaspoon sea salt

- 1/4 teaspoon black pepper

- 1/2 cup canned black beans, rinsed and drained

- 2 tablespoons freshly squeezed lemon juice

- 2 tablespoons freshly chopped parsley

Instructions:

1. Heat oil in a large saucepan over medium-high heat. Add quinoa and cook, stirring often, for 2 minutes.

2. Add vegetable broth and bring to a simmer. Reduce heat to low, cover the pan, and cook for 15 minutes, or until quinoa is tender and liquid is absorbed.

3. Add onion, bell pepper, mushrooms, garlic, oregano, salt, and pepper to the pan and cook for 5 minutes, stirring often.

4. Add black beans to the pan and cook for 2 minutes, stirring often.

5. Drizzle with lemon juice and sprinkle with parsley. Serve immediately.

Ingredients:

- 2 tablespoons olive oil

- 1/2 cup uncooked lentils

- 1 cup vegetable broth

- 1/2 teaspoon dried oregano

- 1/4 teaspoon sea salt

- 1/4 teaspoon black pepper

- 2 cups baby spinach

- 2 tablespoons freshly squeezed lemon juice

- 2 tablespoons freshly chopped parsley

Instructions:

1. Heat oil in a large saucepan over medium-high heat. Add lentils and cook, stirring often, for 2 minutes.

2. Add vegetable broth, oregano, salt, and pepper to the pan and bring to a simmer.

Reduce heat to low, cover the pan, and cook for 10 minutes, or until lentils are tender.

3. Add spinach to the pan and cook for 1 minute, stirring often.

4. Drizzle with lemon juice and sprinkle with parsley. Serve immediately.

Ingredients:

- 2 tablespoons olive oil

- 2 sweet potatoes, cut into 1-inch cubes

- 1/2 teaspoon dried oregano

- 1/4 teaspoon sea salt

- 1/4 teaspoon black pepper

- 1 can chickpeas, rinsed and drained

- 2 tablespoons freshly squeezed lemon juice

- 2 tablespoons freshly chopped parsley

Instructions:

1. Preheat oven to 375 degrees F.

2. Line a baking sheet with parchment paper.

3. Toss sweet potatoes with olive oil, oregano, salt, and pepper. Spread in an even layer on the baking sheet.

4. Roast for 25 minutes, or until sweet potatoes are tender.

5. In a large bowl, combine roasted sweet potatoes, chickpeas, lemon juice, and parsley. Toss to combine.

6. Serve immediately.

Ingredients:

- 2 tablespoons olive oil

- 1 eggplant, diced

- 1/2 teaspoon dried oregano

- 1/4 teaspoon sea salt

- 1/4 teaspoon black pepper

- 1 cup uncooked brown rice

- 2 cups vegetable broth

- 2 tablespoons freshly squeezed lemon juice

- 2 tablespoons freshly chopped parsley

Instructions:

1. Heat oil in a large saucepan over medium-high heat. Add eggplant and cook, stirring often, for 5 minutes.

2. Add oregano, salt, and pepper to the pan and cook for 1 minute, stirring often.

3. Add rice and vegetable broth to the pan and bring to a simmer. Reduce heat to low, cover the pan, and cook for 20 minutes, or until rice is tender and liquid is absorbed.

4. Drizzle with lemon juice and sprinkle with parsley. Serve immediately.

Ingredients:

- 2 tablespoons olive oil

- 1 head of broccoli, cut into florets

- 1/2 teaspoon dried oregano

- 1/4 teaspoon sea salt

- 1/4 teaspoon black pepper

- 1 cup uncooked quinoa

- 2 cups vegetable broth

- 2 tablespoons freshly squeezed lemon juice

- 2 tablespoons freshly chopped parsley

Instructions:

1. Preheat oven to 425 degrees F.

2. Line a baking sheet with parchment paper.

3. Toss broccoli with olive oil, oregano, salt, and pepper. Spread in an even layer on the baking sheet.

4. Roast for 20 minutes, or until broccoli is tender.

5. Heat oil in a large saucepan over medium-high heat. Add quinoa and cook, stirring often, for 2 minutes.

6. Add vegetable broth and bring to a simmer. Reduce heat to low, cover the pan, and cook for 10 minutes, or until quinoa is tender and liquid is absorbed.

7. Add roasted broccoli to the pan and cook for 2 minutes, stirring often.

8. Drizzle with lemon juice and sprinkle with parsley. Serve immediately.

Ingredients:

- 2 tablespoons olive oil

- 1 head of cauliflower, grated

- 1/2 teaspoon chili powder

- 1/4 teaspoon sea salt

- 1/4 teaspoon black pepper

- 1/4 teaspoon smoked paprika

- 1/4 teaspoon garlic powder

- 2 tablespoons freshly squeezed lemon juice

- 2 tablespoons freshly chopped parsley

Instructions:

1. Heat oil in a large skillet over medium-high heat. Add cauliflower and cook, stirring often, for 5 minutes.

2. Add chili powder, salt, pepper, paprika, and garlic powder to the pan and cook for 2 minutes, stirring often.

3. Drizzle with lemon juice and sprinkle with parsley. Serve immediately.

Ingredients:

- 2 tablespoons olive oil

- 1 large zucchini, spiralized

- 1/2 teaspoon dried oregano

- 1/4 teaspoon sea salt

- 1/4 teaspoon black pepper

- 1/4 cup canned black beans, rinsed and drained

- 2 tablespoons freshly squeezed lemon juice

- 2 tablespoons freshly chopped parsley

Instructions:

1. Heat oil in a large skillet over medium-high heat. Add zucchini noodles and cook, stirring often, for 5 minutes.

2. Add oregano, salt, and pepper to the pan and cook for 1 minute, stirring often.

3. Add black beans to the pan and cook for 2 minutes, stirring often.

4. Drizzle with lemon juice and sprinkle with parsley. Serve immediately.

Ingredients:

- 2 tablespoons olive oil

- 1 sweet potato, cut into 1-inch cubes

- 1/2 teaspoon curry powder

- 1/4 teaspoon sea salt

- 1/4 teaspoon black pepper

- 1/2 cup uncooked lentils

- 2 cups vegetable broth

- 2 tablespoons freshly squeezed lemon juice

- 2 tablespoons freshly chopped parsley

Instructions:

1. Preheat oven to 375 degrees F.

2. Line a baking sheet with parchment paper.

3. Toss sweet potatoes with olive oil, curry powder, salt, and pepper. Spread in an even layer on the baking sheet.

4. Roast for 25 minutes, or until sweet potatoes are tender.

5. Heat oil in a large saucepan over medium-high heat. Add lentils and cook, stirring often, for 2 minutes.

6. Add vegetable broth and bring to a simmer. Reduce heat to low, cover the pan, and cook for 10 minutes, or until lentils are tender.

7. Add roasted sweet potatoes to the pan and cook for 2 minutes, stirring often.

8. Drizzle with lemon juice and sprinkle with parsley. Serve immediately.

Ingredients:

- 2 tablespoons olive oil

- 1 eggplant, diced

- 1/2 teaspoon dried oregano

- 1/4 teaspoon sea salt

- 1/4 teaspoon black pepper

- 1 can chickpeas, rinsed and drained

- 2 tablespoons freshly squeezed lemon juice

- 2 tablespoons freshly chopped parsley

Instructions:

1. Preheat oven to 425 degrees F.

2. Line a baking sheet with parchment paper.

3. Toss eggplant with olive oil, oregano, salt, and pepper. Spread in an even layer on the baking sheet.

4. Roast for 20 minutes, or until eggplant is tender.

5. In a large bowl, combine roasted eggplant, chickpeas, lemon juice, and parsley. Toss to combine.

6. Serve immediately.

1. Roasted Salmon and Asparagus (30 minutes)

Ingredients:

- 2 6-ounce salmon fillets

- 2 tablespoons olive oil

- 2 cloves garlic, minced

- 1 tablespoon fresh lemon juice

- 1/2 teaspoon smoked paprika

- 1/4 teaspoon sea salt

- 1/4 teaspoon freshly ground black pepper

- 2 cups asparagus, cut into 1-inch pieces

Instructions:

1. Preheat oven to 400 degrees F.

2. Place salmon fillets in a baking dish.

3. In a small bowl, whisk together olive oil, garlic, lemon juice, paprika, salt, and pepper.

4. Pour mixture over salmon fillets and spread evenly.

5. Place asparagus pieces around the salmon.

6. Bake for 15-20 minutes, or until salmon is cooked through and asparagus is lightly browned.

2. Sautéed Broccoli and Mushrooms (25 minutes)

Ingredients:

- 2 tablespoons olive oil

- 2 cloves garlic, minced

- 1/2 teaspoon sea salt

- 1/4 teaspoon freshly ground black pepper

- 2 cups chopped broccoli

- 1 cup sliced mushrooms

Instructions:

1. Heat oil in a large skillet over medium heat.

2. Add garlic, salt, and pepper and sauté for 1-2 minutes.

3. Add broccoli and mushrooms and sauté for 5-7 minutes, or until vegetables are tender.

Ingredients:

- 2 tablespoons olive oil

- 2 cloves garlic, minced

- 1/2 teaspoon sea salt

- 1/4 teaspoon freshly ground black pepper

- 2 boneless, skinless chicken breasts

- 2 cups sliced bell peppers

- 1 cup sliced zucchini

Instructions:

1. Heat oil in a large skillet over medium heat.

2. Add garlic, salt, and pepper and sauté for 1-2 minutes.

3. Add chicken breasts and cook for 5-7 minutes, or until cooked through.

4. Add bell peppers and zucchini and cook for 3-5 minutes, or until vegetables are tender.

Ingredients:

- 2 6-ounce tilapia fillets

- 2 tablespoons olive oil

- 2 cloves garlic, minced

- 1/2 teaspoon smoked paprika

- 1/4 teaspoon sea salt

- 1/4 teaspoon freshly ground black pepper

- 2 cups chopped broccoli

Instructions:

1. Preheat oven to 400 degrees F.

2. Place tilapia fillets in a baking dish.

3. In a small bowl, whisk together olive oil, garlic, paprika, salt, and pepper.

4. Pour mixture over tilapia fillets and spread evenly.

5. Place broccoli around the tilapia.

6. Bake for 15-20 minutes, or until tilapia is cooked through and broccoli is lightly browned.

Ingredients:

- 2 tablespoons olive oil

- 2 cloves garlic, minced

- 1/2 teaspoon sea salt

- 1/4 teaspoon freshly ground black pepper

- 1 cup cooked quinoa

- 1 cup sliced bell peppers

- 1 cup sliced mushrooms

- 1 cup sliced zucchini

Instructions:

1. Heat oil in a large skillet over medium heat.

2. Add garlic, salt, and pepper and sauté for 1-2 minutes.

3. Add quinoa and vegetables and sauté for 5-7 minutes, or until vegetables are tender.

6. Baked Eggplant and Tomatoes (30 minutes)

Ingredients:

- 2 tablespoons olive oil

- 2 cloves garlic, minced

- 1/2 teaspoon sea salt

- 1/4 teaspoon freshly ground black pepper

- 1 large eggplant, cut into 1-inch cubes

- 1 cup cherry tomatoes

Instructions:

1. Preheat oven to 400 degrees F.

2. Place eggplant cubes in a baking dish.

3. In a small bowl, whisk together olive oil, garlic, salt, and pepper.

4. Pour mixture over eggplant cubes and spread evenly.

5. Place cherry tomatoes around the eggplant.

6. Bake for 15-20 minutes, or until eggplant is tender and tomatoes are lightly browned.

Ingredients:

- 2 tablespoons olive oil

- 2 cloves garlic, minced

- 1/2 teaspoon sea salt

- 1/4 teaspoon freshly ground black pepper

- 1 cup cooked lentils

- 1 cup sliced bell peppers

- 1 cup sliced mushrooms

- 1 cup sliced zucchini

Instructions:

1. Heat oil in a large skillet over medium heat.

2. Add garlic, salt, and pepper and sauté for 1-2 minutes.

3. Add lentils and vegetables and sauté for 5-7 minutes, or until vegetables are tender.

Ingredients:

- 2 sweet potatoes, cut into 1-inch cubes

- 2 tablespoons olive oil

- 2 cloves garlic, minced

- 1/2 teaspoon smoked paprika

- 1/4 teaspoon sea salt

- 1/4 teaspoon freshly ground black pepper

Instructions:

1. Preheat oven to 400 degrees F.

2. Place sweet potato cubes in a baking dish.

3. In a small bowl, whisk together olive oil, garlic, paprika, salt, and pepper.

4. Pour mixture over sweet potato cubes and spread evenly.

5. Bake for 15-20 minutes, or until sweet potatoes are lightly browned.

Ingredients:

- 2 tablespoons olive oil

- 2 cloves garlic, minced

- 1/2 teaspoon sea salt

- 1/4 teaspoon freshly ground black pepper

- 2 zucchini, cut into 1-inch cubes

- 1 cup cherry tomatoes

Instructions:

1. Preheat oven to 400 degrees F.

2. Place zucchini cubes in a baking dish.

3. In a small bowl, whisk together olive oil, garlic, salt, and pepper.

4. Pour mixture over zucchini cubes and spread evenly.

5. Place cherry tomatoes around the zucchini.

6. Bake for 15-20 minutes, or until zucchini is tender and tomatoes are lightly browned.

Ingredients:

- 2 tablespoons olive oil

- 2 cloves garlic, minced

- 1/2 teaspoon sea salt

- 1/4 teaspoon freshly ground black pepper

- 2 cups Brussels sprouts, halved

- 1 cup sliced carrots

Instructions:

1. Preheat oven to 400 degrees F.

2. Place Brussels sprouts and carrots in a baking dish.

3. In a small bowl, whisk together olive oil, garlic, salt, and pepper.

4. Pour mixture over Brussels sprouts and carrots and spread evenly.

5. Bake for 15-20 minutes, or until Brussels sprouts are lightly browned and carrots are tender.

4.4 SNACKS RECIPES

1. Banana and Blueberry Smoothie (10 minutes)

Ingredients:

-1 banana

-1 cup frozen blueberries

-1 cup of low-fat plain yogurt

-2 tablespoons of honey

Instructions:

1. Add the banana, blueberries, yogurt and honey to a blender.

2. Blend the ingredients until they are smooth.

3. Pour the smoothie into a glass and enjoy.

Ingredients:

-2 slices of whole wheat toast

-1/2 avocado

-1 teaspoon of olive oil

-1/4 teaspoon of sea salt

Instructions:

1. Toast the bread and spread the avocado on top.

2. Drizzle the olive oil and sprinkle the sea salt on top.

3. Enjoy.

3. Baked Apples (20 minutes)

Ingredients:

-2 apples

-1 tablespoon of cinnamon

-1 teaspoon of honey

-1 tablespoon of olive oil

Instructions:

1. Preheat the oven to 350 degrees Fahrenheit.

2. Cut the apples into thin slices and place in an oven-safe dish.

3. Drizzle the olive oil, honey, and sprinkle the cinnamon on top.

4. Bake the apples for 20 minutes, until they are soft.

5. Enjoy.

Ingredients:

-1 can of chickpeas

-1 tablespoon of olive oil

-1 teaspoon of garlic powder

-1 teaspoon of paprika

-1/2 teaspoon of sea salt

Instructions:

1. Preheat the oven to 375 degrees Fahrenheit.

2. Drain the chickpeas and pat them dry.

3. Place them on a baking sheet and toss with the olive oil.

4. Sprinkle the garlic powder, paprika and sea salt on top.

5. Roast the chickpeas for 25-30 minutes.

6. Enjoy.

Ingredients:

-1/2 cup of almonds

-1/2 cup of walnuts

-1/2 cup of dried cranberries

-1/2 cup of dried apricots

Instructions:

1. Place the almonds, walnuts, cranberries and apricots in a bowl.

2. Mix all the ingredients together.

3. Enjoy.

Ingredients:

-1/2 cup of hummus

-1 cup of chopped carrots

-1 cup of chopped celery

-1/2 cup of cherry tomatoes

Instructions:

1. Place the hummus in a bowl.

2. Place the chopped carrots, celery and cherry tomatoes in the bowl.

3. Mix all the ingredients together.

4. Enjoy.

Ingredients:

-2 small zucchini

-1/4 cup of almond flour

-1/4 cup of Parmesan cheese

-2 tablespoons of olive oil

-1 teaspoon of garlic powder

-1/2 teaspoon of sea salt

Instructions:

1. Grate the zucchinis and place them in a bowl.

2. Add the almond flour, Parmesan cheese, olive oil, garlic powder and sea salt to the bowl.

3. Mix all the ingredients together.

4. Heat the olive oil in a skillet over medium heat.

5. Form the zucchini mixture into small patties and place them in the skillet.

6. Cook the fritters for 3-4 minutes on each side, until they are golden brown.

7. Enjoy.

Ingredients:

-1 large whole wheat tortilla

-1/4 cup of hummus

-1/2 cup of grated carrots

-1/2 cup of grated cucumber

-1/4 cup of diced tomatoes

Instructions:

1. Spread the hummus on the tortilla.

2. Place the grated carrots, cucumber and tomatoes on top.

3. Roll the tortilla up and cut in half.

4. Enjoy.

Ingredients:

-1/4 cup of chia seeds

-1 cup of almond milk

-2 tablespoons of honey

-1 teaspoon of vanilla extract

-1/4 teaspoon of cinnamon

Instructions:

1. Place the chia seeds in a bowl.

2. Add the almond milk, honey, vanilla extract and cinnamon.

3. Mix all the ingredients together.

4. Refrigerate the mixture for at least 15 minutes, until it is thick and creamy.

5. Enjoy.

Ingredients:

-2 avocados

-1/4 cup of diced tomatoes

-1/4 cup of diced red onion

-2 tablespoons of olive oil

-1/4 teaspoon of sea salt

Instructions:

1. Cut the avocados in half and remove the pit.

2. Place the avocados in an oven-safe dish.

3. Top the avocados with the diced tomatoes and red onion.

4. Drizzle the olive oil and sprinkle the sea salt on top.

5. Bake the avocados for 10 minutes, until they are soft.

6. Enjoy.